THYROGLOSSAL DUCT CYST SURGERY NUTRITION

Complete Guide Unlocking The Secrets Of Nutrition To Rapid Healing After Surgery Success, Nourishing Meal Plans, Recipes, Tips For Optimal Health Wellness

DR. ALLAN FREDA

Contents

Readers of this important guidebook will find a lot of useful information on how to eat properly after surgery for a thyroglossal duct cyst. This book gives people the information they need to make smart decisions about their health and well-being after surgery by looking at how surgical healing affects dietary needs.

Some important parts of this detailed guide are:

1. Understanding Thyroglossal Duct Cyst Surgery: This article shares information about the surgery, such as its goal, possible side effects, and the healing process. People who aren't familiar with medical terms will be able to understand the ideas because they are explained clearly and in everyday language.

2. Nutritional Considerations After Surgery: This book goes into detail about the specific nutrients that are needed for the best healing after surgery for a thyroglossal duct cyst.

It gives evidence-based advice on the nutrients that are needed for recovery. From protein to vitamins and minerals, readers will learn how to make their food work best for them while they heal.

3. Spiritual Healing Recipes and Meal Plans: This part combines the useful with the tasty. It has a collection of healing recipes that are good for you and taste great. Each meal is made with nutrition after surgery in mind, from hearty soups to smoothies full of good things for you.

Customizable meal plans also give people who are trying to figure out their dietary needs during recovery order ease.

4. Tips from Health Professionals for Long-Term Wellness: This guide uses the knowledge of health professionals to give you great advice on how to stay healthy after surgery and beyond. People who read this will learn how to make changes to their

food, lifestyle, and ongoing self-care habits that will support their long-term health.

This book is a must-have for anyone starting their healing from thyroglossal duct cyst surgery because it covers everything you need to know about nutrition after surgery. "Optimal Nutrition After Thyroglossal Duct Cyst Surgery" gives you the information and tools you need to put your health first and do well in the days and years to come, whether you've just been diagnosed or are helping a loved one through the process.

INTRODUCTION

Thyroglossal duct cyst surgery is often used to get rid of a cyst or mass that forms from the remains of the thyroglossal duct while the embryo is still developing. Surgery removes the cyst completely, but good nutrition is also very important for speeding up the healing process and maintaining general health. In this in-depth guide, we talk about how important diet is for healing after surgery for a thyroglossal duct cyst.

We'll talk about the important nutrients you need for healing, possible food choices, healing recipes, meal plans, and fitness tips from experts for long-term health.

How to Know How Important Food Is for Recovery:

Nutrition is an important part of care after surgery because it has a direct effect on how well the body heals and recovers. After treatment to remove a thyroglossal duct cyst, the body needs a lot of nutrients to help tissues heal, boost the immune system, and lower the risk of complications.

 A healthy diet full of important minerals, vitamins, protein, and antioxidants is important for wound healing, lowering inflammation, and getting strength and energy back. Good nutrition not only speeds up the healing process but also improves health and well-being in the long run.

A full guide to the best diet for people who have just had surgery or been diagnosed with a new illness.

It includes healing recipes, meal plans, and expert advice for long-term health:

Important Nutrients for Healing:

After surgery to remove a thyroglossal duct cyst, the body may need more nutrients to help it heal. Protein, vitamins, minerals, and antioxidants are some of the most important foods for repairing tissues, boosting the immune system, and lowering inflammation.

Protein is very important for wound healing and tissue repair because it gives new cells and tissues the building blocks they need to grow. Lean protein sources, like chicken, fish, tofu, beans, and dairy products, must be included in the diet to meet protein needs after surgery. Vitamins C, E, zinc, and omega-3 fatty acids can also help the body heal and reduce problems after surgery because they are antioxidants and anti-inflammatory. Eating a range of fruits, vegetables, whole grains, nuts, and seeds will help you get enough of these important nutrients.

A healthy, well-balanced diet is important for overall recovery, but there are some things people should remember about their food after surgery for a thyroglossal duct cyst. Staying hydrated means having a lot of water throughout the day.

Staying hydrated is important for healing tissues and staying healthy in general. Eating small meals more often can also help you feel better and stop you from feeling sick, especially right after surgery.

It is also suggested that you stay away from foods that are high in sugar, sodium, and bad fats since these can make the inflammation worse and slow down the healing process. Instead, focus on eating foods that are high in nutrients, like fruits, vegetables, lean proteins, whole grains, and healthy fats, to help your body heal and stay healthy in the long run.

Adding healing meals to your diet after surgery can help you eat healthy, nutrient-dense foods that will help you heal and feel better overall.

Here are some easy meals that are also good for you:

1. Healing Chicken Vegetable Soup: This hearty soup is full of healthy fats from the chicken and vitamins and minerals from the different veggies.

In a pot, mix diced chicken breast, carrots, celery, onion, garlic, and low-sodium chicken broth. Cook until the vegetables are tender.

Add your favorite herbs and spices to make it taste better.

2. Quinoa salad with roasted veggies: Quinoa is a complete protein that gives your body the amino acids it needs to repair tissue. Roasted vegetables

like bell peppers, zucchini, and cherry tomatoes add vitamins, minerals, and antioxidants to the salad.

Add cooked quinoa to roasted veggies, olive oil, lemon juice, and fresh herbs to make a salad that is both healthy and filling.

3. Baked salmon with steamed asparagus: Salmon is high in omega-3 fatty acids, which help the body heal after surgery by reducing inflammation. For an easy but healthy meal that is high in protein, vitamins, and minerals, serve baked salmon with steamed asparagus.

4. Greek Yoghurt Parfait with Berries and Almonds: Greek yogurt is a great way to get protein and probiotics, which are good for your immune system and gut health.

You can make a tasty and healthy parfait by layering Greek yogurt with mixed berries and nuts. This parfait is great for breakfast or as a healthy snack.

Making a well-balanced meal plan is important to make sure you get all the nutrients you need while you are healing from thyroglossal duct cyst surgery. Here is an example of a meal plan to help you:

• Over easy eggs with spinach and whole grain toast for breakfast

• Snack in the middle of the morning: Greek yogurt with honey and mixed veggies

• Lunch: mixed veggies, grilled chicken breast, and quinoa salad

A snack in the afternoon would be hummus with sliced veggies.

• For dinner, I made baked salmon with rice pilaf and steamed broccoli.

• Snack in the evening: cottage cheese with pineapple chunks

It's important to pay attention to your body and make changes to your meal plan as needed based on your specific food needs and tastes.

In addition to paying attention to what you eat right after surgery, making healthy lifestyle choices can help you stay healthy in the long run and stop thyroglossal duct cysts from coming back. Check out these tips from experts:

1. Stay Active: Regular exercise not only improves your health and well-being, but it also helps you recover from surgery more quickly. Your goal should be to do at least 30 minutes of moderately intense exercise most days of the week. Some examples of this would be walking, swimming, or riding.

2. Control your stress: Long-term stress can hurt your immune system and make it harder to heal. To relax and feel less stressed, try stress-relieving

activities like tai chi, yoga, meditation, or deep breathing routines.

3. Follow Up with Your Healthcare Provider: Keep your follow-up meetings with your healthcare provider to make sure you're getting better and to talk about any worries or problems that may come up.

4. Quit smoking. Smoking can slow the healing of wounds and raise the risk of problems after surgery. If you smoke, you might want to quit or get help to do it for good.

5. Maintain a Healthy Weight: Eating well and working out regularly can help you reach and stay at a healthy weight, which can lower your risk of health problems and improve your general health.

Focusing on nutrition and using these expert tips as part of your post-surgery care plan can help you recover fully from thyroglossal duct cyst surgery and improve your health and well-being in the long run.

CHAPTER 1
GETTING READY FOR SURGERY

There is more to getting ready for surgery than just making an appointment and showing up on the day of the process. It requires a complete plan that includes getting ready mentally and physically and thinking about what to eat. One popular surgery is thyroglossal duct cyst surgery, which is meant to get rid of a cyst or mass that forms along the path of the thyroid gland when an embryo is growing.

To get the best results from this surgery and make healing easier afterward, you need to carefully prepare. Nutrition is an important part of getting ready because it helps the body heal. This guide will go over the most important nutritional things you should think about before having surgery for a thyroglossal duct cyst.

It will focus on pre-surgery nutrition basics and making your home a healing space.

What you eat is very important for getting your body ready for surgery. A healthy, well-balanced diet full of important nutrients not only helps the body fix itself better, but also boosts the immune system, lowers the risk of complications, and speeds up the healing process. Before thyroglossal duct cyst surgery, it's important to eat a lot of nutrient-dense foods that are good for your general health and help your body handle the stress of surgery. Some important things to think about when it comes to diet before surgery:

1. Maintain Adequate Hydration: Staying properly hydrated is important for your health and the best possible result of surgery. To stay refreshed in the days before the surgery, try to drink a lot of water and other fluids.

Avoid drinking too much alcohol and caffeine drinks because they can make you lose water.

2. Pay attention to whole foods: Choose whole, raw foods that are high in antioxidants, phytonutrients, vitamins, and minerals. In your diet, eat a lot of fruits, veggies, whole grains, lean proteins, and healthy fats. These foods give you important nutrients that help your immune system work, tissues heal, and your general health.

3. Protein is important for repairing tissues and treating wounds, so you need to eat more of it before and after surgery. When you eat, try to include protein-rich foods like chicken, fish, eggs, dairy, nuts, seeds, and beans. Aim for a healthy amount of protein throughout the day to keep your muscles strong and help them heal.

4. Increase your intake of antioxidants. Antioxidants fight oxidative stress, lower inflammation, and help the immune system work better, all of which are important for healing.

Eat a wide range of antioxidant-rich foods, like nuts, seeds, citrus fruits, leafy greens, cruciferous veggies, berries, and spices.

5. Make sure you get enough micronutrients. Vitamins and minerals are important for many bodily functions, such as immune system function, collagen production, and tissue repair. To help your health and healing, eat foods that are high in zinc, selenium, magnesium, iron, vitamins A, C, D, and E, as well as B vitamins.

6. Limit processed foods and sugary snacks: These foods aren't very good for you and can slow down your mending process. Eat less processed foods, sugary snacks, refined carbohydrates, and unhealthy fats. Choose whole foods that are high in nutrients to properly feed your body.

7. Talk to a trained Dietitian: If you are worried about certain foods or have a health problem that could affect your nutrition, you might want to talk to a trained dietitian or nutritionist.

They can give you personalized advice and suggestions that are made to fit your specific needs, making sure that you're well-fed before surgery.

By paying attention to these pre-surgery nutrition basics, you can improve your general health, make sure you have the best nutrition, and speed up the healing process for your thyroglossal duct cyst.

As a bonus, making your kitchen a healing space can help you get ready for surgery and set you up for a quick recovery.

How to Make Your Kitchen a Healing Space

The kitchen is the heart of the home because it's where food is made, people are fed, and healing starts. It takes more than stocking up on healthy foods to make your kitchen a healing space. It's about making it a place that encourages health, wellness, and thoughtful eating. Here are some ways to make your kitchen a healing space, whether you're getting ready for surgery or just thinking about your long-term health:

1. Stock up on Nutrient-Dense Foods: Put a range of nutrient-dense foods that are good for your health and healing in your kitchen. It's important to have fresh fruits and veggies, whole grains, lean proteins, healthy fats, and pantry staples like nuts, seeds, beans, lentils, whole grain pasta, quinoa, and whole grain pasta. When you don't have much time, it's easier to make healthy meals and snacks when your kitchen is well-stocked.

2. Streamline Your Kitchen Layout and Organization: Streamlining your kitchen layout and organization will make cooking faster and more fun. Keep pots, pans, and tools that you use often close at hand, and set aside areas for preparing meals, cooking, and storing things. Clear off the counters to make a clean, welcoming place for cooking and eating that encourages mindfulness.

3. Prioritise Food Safety and Hygiene: Keep food safety and hygiene standards high to avoid getting sick from food and to support good health. Before touching food, wash your hands well. Regularly clean and sanitize cooking surfaces. Store perishable foods at the right temperatures to keep them from going bad. To keep raw meat, chicken, and seafood from getting contaminated with each other, use different cutting boards and tools for each.

4. Create a Calm Environment: Make your kitchen a calm, peaceful place that encourages you to relax and eat mindfully. To make a space feel calm, play relaxing music, light candles, or add natural elements like plants or flowers. Keep things like TV and electronics out of the way as much as possible so you can fully concentrate on cooking and enjoying your meals.

5. Try Healing Recipes and Meal Plans: Look for new recipes and meal ideas that focus on whole,

healthy foods that are known to have healing qualities. To help your body heal itself, eat foods that reduce inflammation, ingredients that boost your immune system, and superfoods that are high in nutrients. Try different herbs, spices, and cooking methods to make your meals taste better and be more interesting while also getting the most nutritional value out of them.

6. Mindful Eating: To practice mindful eating, pay attention to your body's signals for when it's hungry and when it's full, savor each bite, and eat with purpose and gratitude. You should try to avoid electronic gadgets and TV during meals as much as possible. Instead, enjoy the tastes, textures, and smells of your food. Mindful eating can help your body digest food better, make you feel full, and connect you more deeply with your food and body.

7. Include loved ones in meal preparation: Whether it's family, friends, or carers, include

loved ones in meal preparation to make it a fun activity to do together. Together cooking not only brings people and lets them get to know each other better, but it also gives you the chance to share the joy of feeding others home-cooked meals made with love and care. To build a sense of empowerment and teamwork, get everyone involved in planning meals, going food shopping, and cooking.

By turning your kitchen into a healing space, you can help yourself get ready for surgery, recover from surgery, and stay healthy in the long run.

You can make your kitchen a place of health, healing, and nourishment by focusing on nutrient-dense foods, organizing it so it's easy to use, putting food safety and hygiene first, making it a relaxing space, trying out healing recipes and meal plans, practicing mindful eating, and getting your family involved in making meals. Your kitchen can be a very helpful place to help you get healthy and heal, whether you're about to have surgery or just want to be as healthy as possible.

CHAPTER 2
HEALTHY RECOVERY RECIPES

For people who have recently had surgery, like thyroglossal duct cyst surgery, what they eat is very important for their recovery. During recovery, the body needs more nutrients than usual because it needs to repair tissues, improve the immune system, and get stronger. This complete guide to the best post-surgery diet for people who have just been found with thyroglossal duct cysts goes into detail about how important it is to stay healthy while you're healing. It includes meal plans, healing recipes, and expert advice for long-term health.

Why post-surgery nutrition is important

When you have surgery to remove a thyroglossal duct cyst, your body goes through a lot of changes that need a good diet for the best healing and recovery. A good diet not only helps wounds heal faster, but it also helps fight complications after surgery, like infections and taking too long to recover. Eating foods that are high in nutrients is important for rebuilding cells, getting energy back, and helping the immune system. This makes sure that the healing process goes smoothly and effectively.

Soups are great for people who have had surgery to remove a thyroglossal duct cyst because they keep you warm, keep you hydrated, and provide nutrients that are easy to digest.

Choose vegetable soups or broths that you make yourself. Carrots, celery, ginger, and garlic are all healthy foods that you can add to these soups.

You can make soups even healthier by adding protein sources like chicken or lentils. Protein helps fix tissues and build muscle. Pureeing foods until they are smooth can also help with swallowing, making them perfect for people who are in pain or having trouble chewing after surgery.

Pureed foods are easy on the throat and swallow, so people with thyroglossal duct cysts need to make sure they have them on their diet after surgery.

By blending soft foods like cooked fruits, veggies, beans, and tofu, you can make healthy purees that are full of the vitamins, minerals, and antioxidants your body needs to heal. Try out different flavor blends and textures to keep meals interesting and tasty. Adding healthy fats like olive oil or avocado to purees can make them higher in calories and make you feel full, which can help you keep your weight steady while you recover.

People who are healing from surgery for a thyroglossal duct cyst can easily get a nutritious meal or snack in the form of smoothies or shakes.

You can make tasty drinks that are full of vitamins, minerals, and protein by blending different fruits, leafy veggies, yogurt, nut butter, and protein powder.

Adding flaxseeds, chia seeds, or hemp hearts to smoothies can make them higher in fiber and omega-3 fatty acids, which are good for your gut health and reduce inflammation. Adding vitamin C-rich foods, like citrus fruits or berries, can also help the immune system work better and speed up the healing of wounds.

Soups and teas made from herbs that heal

Along with eating solid foods, keeping hydrated is very important for helping your body heal and improving your overall health after thyroglossal duct cyst surgery. Healing broths and plant teas can help you stay hydrated and give you good nutrients and antioxidants. In particular, bone broth is full of vitamins, amino acids, and collagen that help keep your gut healthy, your joints working well, and your skin flexible. Anti-inflammatory plants like turmeric, ginger, and chamomile can be added to herbal teas to help with pain and stress after surgery. Staying hydrated is important to avoid problems like diarrhea and urinary tract infections that are common after surgery.

Optimizing diet after surgery is very important for people who have had thyroglossal duct cyst surgery. People can help their bodies heal and stay healthy for a long time by focusing on nutrient-dense foods and drinks like healing broths, warming soups, soft purees, and smoothies high in nutrients. People can feel more confident in their recovery process and make sure they have a smooth return to good health by trying out different recipes, meal plans, and expert tips.

CHAPTER 3
DELICIES THAT CHANGE THE TEXTURE

When you have surgery for a thyroglossal duct cyst, good nutrition is very important for your healing and general recovery. It's important to pay close attention to what you eat after surgery to help tissues heal, lower inflammation, and boost your immune system. Understanding the importance of texture-changed treats, soft and tender protein meals, flavorful mashed creations, and filling porridges and congees is a big part of getting the right nutrition after surgery. People who have had surgery to remove a thyroglossal duct cyst can choose from a variety of foods in these categories that are specifically designed to meet their needs. These foods will help them get all the nutrients they need while also making processing easier and reducing pain.

When you are right after surgery for a thyroglossal duct cyst, the taste of your food is very important. Because tissues in the throat are moved around during surgery, patients often feel pain or have trouble swallowing.

Texture-modified delights are an answer because they offer healthy options that are easy on the throat and full of important nutrients. There is a wide range of textures in these treats, from soft and tender to smooth and creamy, so everyone can find something that suits their tastes and comfort levels.

Protein dishes that are soft and tender:

Protein is a necessary nutrient for muscle repair and regeneration, which makes it very important after surgery. But because they are tough or chewy, standard protein sources may be hard for people who have had surgery to remove a thyroglossal duct cyst. Protein dishes that are soft and tender are an option.

They provide enough protein without making you chew or swallow a lot. Poached or shredded chicken, tender fish pieces, scrambled eggs, and tofu made softly are all examples of this type of food. Not only do these choices provide important amino acids for healing, but they are also easy to eat and digest, which also helps with recovery.

Delicious Mashed Recipes:

Another important food for people with thyroglossal duct cysts to eat after surgery is mashed foods. Not only does mashing soften foods, but it also makes them taste better and makes them easier to swallow and digest.

You can mash a lot of different things together, like fruits, veggies, grains, and legumes, to make a wide range of tasty and healthy foods. Mashed potatoes, sweet potato mash, mashed avocado, pumpkin puree, and mashed banana are all tasty examples of mashed foods. By using healthy fats like olive oil, avocado, herbs, and spices, these recipes can be both tasty and good for you, helping you heal and get better after surgery.

Porridges and congees that fill you up:
Porridges and congees are soothing and healthy foods that are great for people who have recently had surgery to remove a thyroglossal duct cyst. These meals are made with grains or rice that have been cooked until they are soft and mushy.

They are often served with broth or milk to add flavour and moisture. Porridges and congees are warm and welcoming, and they provide energy-giving carbs and fiber that are good for your digestive system. You can add different things to them, like veggies, lean proteins, and herbs, to make them taste better and be healthier. Some examples are oatmeal porridge, rice congee, barley porridge, and quinoa porridge. All of these are filling and easy-to-digest meals that can help you heal from surgery.

A Complete Guide to the Best Post-Surgery Diet for People Who Have Just Been Diagnosed, With Healing Recipes, Meal Plans, and Wellness Tips from Experts for Long-Term Health:

Adopting the best post-surgery food is very important for speeding up recovery, avoiding complications, and maintaining long-term health after thyroglossal duct cyst surgery.

This detailed guide is meant to help people who have just been told they have thyroglossal duct cysts figure out what they need to eat after surgery. With healing recipes, meal plans, and expert advice, this guide gives you useful ways to improve your nutrition and health while you're recovering and afterward.

Recipes for Healing:

Healing recipes are the basis of a good post-surgery diet because they provide tasty and healthy choices that are specifically designed to help with healing and tissue repair.

These recipes focus on using foods that are high in nutrients and provide the vitamins, minerals, and antioxidants that the body needs to heal.

Healing recipes include a range of whole foods, such as fruits, vegetables, lean proteins, whole grains, and healthy fats. They provide a balanced approach to nutrition while also accommodating different dietary needs and tastes. Soups, stews, smoothies, salads, and grain bowls are all examples of healing recipes. Each one is made to provide a powerful mix of nutrients and flavors to help with recovery from surgery and general health.

Planned meals:

People who have thyroglossal duct cysts can incorporate healthy eating into their daily lives after surgery with the help of structured meal plans. The goal of these meal plans is to make sure that you get the right amount of macronutrients (like carbs, proteins, and fats) and micronutrients (like vitamins and minerals) to help your body heal and stay healthy.

Individuals can have meal plans that are made just for them, taking into account things like age, gender, level of exercise, and food preferences. They advise on food choices, portion sizes, and when to eat to help people get the most nutrients while minimizing pain and improving digestive health during the recovery time.

Long-Term Health Tips from Experts:

People who have had surgery to remove a thyroglossal duct cyst need more than just recovery recipes and meal plans. They also need to include expert tips for long-term health. There are many ways to improve your nutrition, deal with symptoms, and improve your general health that aren't just for the first few days after surgery. Staying hydrated, eating a wide range of colorful fruits and vegetables, practicing mindful eating, getting regular exercise, and getting help from healthcare professionals like registered dietitians or nutritionists for personalized guidance and advice are all examples of expert tips. People who follow these expert tips can set themselves up for long-term health and wellness after surgery for a thyroglossal duct cyst. This will make the shift to a thriving life after surgery go more smoothly.

CHAPTER 4
TASTEFUL BLENDED MEALS

Surgery to remove a thyroglossal duct cyst is usually beneficial, but it can be a big event in a person's life, especially when it comes to recovery and care after surgery.

During the recovery time, nutrition is very important because it helps wounds heal, boosts the immune system, and makes sure everyone is healthy overall. People who have had surgery may feel pain or have trouble swallowing, which can make it hard for them to eat solid things. In these situations, tasty mixed meals can be an easy and healthy way to meet the body's nutritional needs.

Blended meals that taste great:

Blended meals are great for people who have had surgery to remove a thyroglossal duct cyst because they have a smooth texture that makes them easier to swallow and digest.

These meals can be changed to include different nutrient-dense foods, making sure that patients get all the vitamins, minerals, and protein they need to heal properly. Also, blended meals are flexible and can be changed to fit different dietary needs and tastes.

After surgery, healthy and filling blended bowls are a good choice for food. Usually, these bowls have a base, like cooked grains or legumes, that are mixed with fruits, veggies, and protein sources.

 Leafy veggies, avocados, berries, tofu, and lean meats are all common ingredients.

Wholesome blended bowls provide a complete nutritional profile by using a variety of vegetables that provide important nutrients such as antioxidants, vitamins, minerals, fiber, and more. Besides that, they give you steady energy to help your body heal and improve your general health.

Creamy mixed soups are another tasty and healthy option for people who have recently had surgery to remove a thyroglossal duct cyst.

You make these soups by pureeing cooked veggies, broth, and other things together until the soup is smooth and creamy. Butternut squash soup, creamy tomato soup, and broccoli and cheese soup are all popular choices.

Not only are blended soups easy to take, but they are also good for people who are having trouble eating because they are soothing to the throat.

They can also be made stronger by adding protein-rich foods like Greek yogurt, beans, or lentils to help muscles heal and mend.

Smoothie bowls full of nutrients:

After surgery, smoothie bowls are a relaxing and nutrient-dense way to eat, especially for people who may have trouble chewing or swallowing solid foods. A thick and creamy smoothie base made from blended fruits, veggies, and liquids like milk or yogurt is often found in these bowls.

Toppings like fresh fruit pieces, granola, nuts, and seeds give the cereal more texture, flavor, and nutrients. Patients can add ingredients that meet their specific dietary needs and tastes to smoothie bowls because they are very flexible. They have a lot of antioxidants, vitamins, minerals, fiber, and fiber, which help the immune system work and speed up recovery from surgery.

A full guide to the best diet for people who have just had surgery or been diagnosed with a new illness. It includes healing recipes, meal plans, and expert advice for long-term health:

Adopting the best post-surgery food is important for helping with recovery and promoting long-term health after thyroglossal duct cyst surgery.

This complete guide gives readers useful information, healthy recipes, meal plans, and expert advice to help them meet their nutritional needs.

Healing recipes are carefully made to give the body the nutrients it needs to heal and get better after surgery. These recipes focus on using foods that are high in nutrients and known to help with healing, like fruits, veggies, whole grains, lean proteins, and healthy fats.

Smoothies that are high in antioxidants, quinoa salads that are high in protein, comforting vegetable soups, and nourishing Buddha bowls are all examples of healing meals. People can speed up the healing process, lower inflammation, and improve their general health by adding these healing recipes to their diet.

Making organized meal plans can help people who have had surgery for a thyroglossal duct cyst make sure they always get the nutrients they need.

Fruits, veggies, whole grains, lean proteins, and healthy fats are just a few of the nutrient-dense foods that should be in a well-balanced meal plan. For each person, meal plans should also include their calorie and nutrient needs as well as any food restrictions or tastes. By following a personalized meal plan, people can get the most out of their food, speed up the healing process, and keep their energy up while they're recovering.

Tips from experts for long-term health:

Along with healing recipes and meal plans, adding long-term health tips from experts can help people on their nutrition journey after surgery even more. Some of these tips might be ways to deal with common side effects of surgery, like pain, swelling, or trouble eating.

They might also include suggestions for making exercise a part of daily life to improve health and well-being in general.

Experts may also advise on how to eat mindfully, control portions, and keep a varied diet to help with long-term weight management and avoid nutritional deficiencies. People can form healthy habits that will improve their health and quality of life after recovery time by using these expert tips in their daily lives.

CHAPTER 5

MEALS THAT ARE EASY TO EAT

Some surgeries, especially ones that are done on sensitive areas like the neck, can make it very hard to eat afterward.

This is especially important for people who have had surgery for a thyroglossal duct cyst because they need to be careful about what they eat while they heal.

Choosing meals that are easy to swallow is very important during this time to make sure you get enough nutrition while minimizing pain.

These foods are made to be easy on the throat, esophagus, and muscles nearby, which helps the body heal and improves health in general.

Casseroles and bakes that are tender

People who have recently had surgery to remove a thyroglossal cyst should eat tender casseroles and bakes.

Most of the time, these meals have cooked, soft ingredients that don't need to be chewed much, so they're easy to swallow. Casseroles often have a lot of healthy foods in them, like veggies, lean proteins, and grains. This makes for a well-rounded meal that helps with healing and recovery.

When you bake these ingredients together, the flavors blend and the textures get softer. The result is a warming dish that is easy on the stomach and throat. Also, casseroles can be made ahead of time and heated up when needed, which is helpful for people who are dealing with the challenges of healing after surgery.

Meatloafs that are moist and tasty

Meatloaf is a standard comfort food that can be changed to fit the needs of people who have had surgery to remove a thyroglossal duct cyst.

Meatloaf is easier to swallow when it is made with lean ground meats and lots of ingredients that are high in water, like veggies or breadcrumbs that have been soaked in broth. Adding tasty herbs, spices, and sauces like tomato or mushroom gravy to meatloaf can make it both healthy and filling, giving you the nutrients you need and helping your body heal. By cutting meatloaf into small, bite-sized pieces, you make it even better for people who have trouble eating, making it easier to eat and enjoy.

Delicate dishes made with fish and seafood

Fish and fish are good for you in many ways.

They contain high-quality protein, omega-3 fatty acids, and many vitamins and minerals. People who have had surgery to remove a thyroglossal duct cyst may find that eating delicate fish and seafood dishes is both good for them and fun. Lean protein can be found in foods like baked salmon pieces, poached white fish, or prawn stir-fries that don't require a lot of chewing.

By using gentle cooking methods like baking, steaming, or poaching, these seafood choices keep the soft texture that makes them easy to swallow. This makes eating them less painful.

Adding flavorful herbs, citrus, or light sauces can also improve the taste of these foods, making them appealing to people whose taste buds have changed after surgery.

This is a complete guide to the best diet for people who have just been diagnosed with cancer. It includes healing recipes, meal plans, and expert tips for long-term health.

After surgery for a thyroglossal duct cyst, it is important to eat a diet that is high in nutrients to help the body heal and stay healthy in the long run. This complete guide has helpful information on how to make the best diet after surgery.

It has healing recipes, customisable meal plans, and expert advice to make the recovery process go smoothly.

Recipes for Healing

Healing recipes are very important for diet after surgery because they focus on using ingredients that help tissues heal, lower inflammation, and boost the immune system.

Eating foods that are high in nutrients, like fruits, veggies, whole grains, lean proteins, and healthy fats, can help your body get the vitamins, minerals, and antioxidants it needs to heal properly. Soups, smoothies, and salads that are high in protein, nutrients, and other good things for you can be made in a variety of ways to suit everyone's tastes and nutritional needs. Adding ingredients that are known to help heal, like ginger, turmeric, garlic, and leafy greens, can make these recipes even more therapeutic, helping people get better faster and improving their general health.

Plans for meals

Building regular meal plans into your routine is a good way to make sure you get enough nutrients and help your body heal after surgery.

These meal plans can be changed to fit each person's dietary needs, preferences, and any special instructions from their healthcare providers.

Meal plans can help keep your energy up, help your muscles heal, and keep you from falling short on nutrients by including foods from different food groups and making sure that the amounts of carbs, proteins, and fats are balanced.

Also, eating smaller meals and snacks more often can help your body handle food and absorb nutrients better, which is good for your health and well-being while you're recovering.

When making meal plans, it's important to be flexible and adaptable so that they can be changed based on hunger, tolerance, and any changing dietary needs as healing goes on.

In addition to focusing on nutrition right after surgery, it is also important to put long-term health first to improve health results and avoid future problems. Healthcare workers, nutritionists, and other experts can give you useful advice on how to keep living a healthy life after you've recovered.

As an example, these tips might include getting regular exercise, dealing with worry, drinking plenty of water, and eating mindfully. Also, keeping an eye on your nutrition, making regular follow-up visits with your healthcare providers, and being honest about any worries or problems you're having can help you stay on track and be healthy for a long time. People can not only recover from surgery but also improve their health and well-being for years to come by following these expert suggestions and making changes to their lifestyle that will last.

CHAPTER 6
SNACKS AND TREATS THAT ARE GOOD FOR YOU

Eating right is very important for getting better after having surgery on your thyroid, especially to remove a thyroglossal duct cyst. A healthy, well-balanced diet not only helps wounds heal but also keeps you healthy and full of energy.

This detailed guide talks about how healing snacks and treats like energy bites, soft cookies, and smooth puddings can help with the best recovery and long-term health.

Energy Bites and Bars That Are Good for You

Energy bites and bars are easy to carry and full of nutrients, making them perfect for people who are recovering from surgery. With their healthy ingredients and small size, these treats give you a steady energy boost without making your blood sugar levels rise.

When you make energy bites, choose foods that are high in protein, healthy fats, fiber, vitamins, and minerals. Adding things like nuts, seeds, oats, dried fruits, and nut butter to these snacks not only makes them taste better but also makes them healthier.

And to help the body heal, think about adding things like turmeric or ginger that have anti-inflammatory qualities. Using similar ingredients, you can make energy bars that are easy to eat by pressing them into a bar shape. Energy bites and bars are a healthy way to get fuel for recovery and general well-being after surgery. They can be eaten as a quick pick-me-up between meals or as a snack before a workout.

Cookies that are soft and chewy are a warm and indulgent treat that is also good for you after surgery. By changing some things about traditional cookie recipes, you can make tasty, healthy choices that help the healing process.

When making soft cookies to eat after surgery, you might want to use items that are easy on the stomach and help the body heal. Whole grain flours, like wheat or almond flour, have complex carbs and fiber that give you the energy that lasts and helps your digestive system work better.

Adding things like mashed bananas or applesauce can give the cookies natural sweetness and moisture, so you don't have to use as many refined sugars and bad fats. Adding things like dark chocolate chips, nuts, or seeds not only makes the food taste better but also adds healthy nutrients like omega-3 fatty acids and vitamins.

Soft and chewy cookies are a satisfying treat that can be eaten as a snack or dessert.

They also help with healing and make it easier to stick to a healthy diet after surgery.

Puddings and custards that are smooth

Smooth puddings and custards are a creamy and decadent choice for people who want to eat something comforting and healthy after surgery. The soft texture of these treats makes them easy to take and gentle on the throat, making them great for people who are hurting or having trouble chewing after surgery.

When making smooth puddings and custards, it's important to use ingredients that are good for you and add flavor. As the base for the custard or custard, use healthy ingredients like low-fat milk or plant-based milk like almond milk or coconut milk. Adding things like pureed fruits or veggies not only makes the dish taste better, but also gives it the vitamins, minerals, and antioxidants that it needs. Honey or maple syrup are natural sweeteners that can be used in small amounts to add sweetness without overpowering the flavors of the other ingredients. Add chia seeds or ground flaxseeds, which are high in fiber, protein, and healthy fats, to make the recipe even healthier.

Smooth puddings and custards are a tasty and healthy choice for people recovering from thyroid surgery.

They can be eaten on their own as a snack or as part of a balanced meal. This can help with healing and long-term health.

CHAPTER 7
GETTING STRONG AGAIN

To help you heal and get stronger after having thyroid surgery, especially thyroglossal duct cyst surgery, you need to eat in a variety of ways.

Good nutrition is an important part of healing because it helps with tissue repair, immune system function, and general health. When you have surgery, your body goes through changes that require you to get enough nutrients to help you heal and stay healthy.

Meals Full of Protein to Help You Get Better:

Protein is an important part of the diet after surgery because it helps repair tissues and build muscle. Adding meals that are high in protein can help the body heal faster and get stronger again.

Choose protein foods that are low in fat, like chicken, fish, eggs, tofu, beans, and low-fat dairy.

These foods give your body the important amino acids it needs to make collagen and heal damaged tissues. Protein-rich foods should be a part of every meal and snack to make sure you get enough nutrients to help you heal and keep your muscles from losing mass.

Eating meals that are high in protein can also help control your appetite and make you feel full, which is especially helpful during the recovery time when your appetite may change. Including different types of protein in your diet will make sure you get all the nutrients you need for full healing. You might also want to add protein pills or shakes if it's hard to get enough protein from whole foods alone, especially for people who need more protein because they had surgery.

Getting Stronger with Nutrient-Dense Foods:
Along with protein, foods that are high in vitamins, minerals, and enzymes are also very important for building strength after surgery.

These foods give your body the nutrients it needs to keep your immune system working well, heal damaged tissues, and stay healthy generally. Eating a wide range of fruits, veggies, whole grains, nuts, and seeds will make sure you get all the micronutrients you need for a quick recovery.

Vitamins C and E are found in large amounts in fruits and veggies. These vitamins are antioxidants, which help reduce swelling and speed up the healing process. Whole grains have complex carbohydrates that your body needs to make energy, and nuts and seeds have healthy fats that your body needs to make hormones and keep cell membranes strong. Adding a variety of nutrient-dense foods to your diet is good for your health in general and helps you heal after surgery.

Also, keeping hydrated is important for recovery because it helps move nutrients around, get rid of waste, and keep tissues moist. Aim to drink a lot of water throughout the day, and think about adding foods that are high in water, like fruits and veggies, to your meals and snacks. Avoid drinks with a lot of sugar and caffeine because they can make you dehydrated and slow down the healing process.

getting stronger after surgery for a thyroglossal duct cyst takes a healthy, well-balanced diet that helps repair tissues, build muscles, and improve overall health. Focus on eating meals that are high in protein and nutrients to help your body heal and stay healthy in the long run. Talking to a doctor or registered dietitian about your nutrition needs and tastes is the best way to get personalized advice.

A full guide to the best diet for people who have just had surgery or been diagnosed with a new illness. It includes healing recipes, meal plans, and expert advice for long-term health:

Getting through the time after surgery can be hard, but if you make healthy choices about what you eat and how you live, you can speed up your recovery and improve your health in the long run.

There are healing recipes, meal plans, and expert health tips in this complete guide that will help you make the most of your food after surgery.

It is very important to know how nutrition affects the mending process so that you can heal faster and get stronger after surgery. A healthy meal full of protein, vitamins, minerals, and antioxidants gives your body the nutrients it needs to repair tissues, keep your immune system strong, and stay healthy overall. Focusing on nutrient-dense foods and developing healing recipes in your weekly meal plans can help your body heal and improve your overall health.

Healing recipes are carefully made to give you a mix of nutrients that help you get better and heal faster. Protein-, vitamin-, and mineral-dense foods like lean meats, fish, poultry, fruits, veggies, whole grains, nuts, and seeds are often used in these recipes. By including healing recipes in your meal plans, you can be sure that your body is getting all the nutrients it needs to get stronger and stay healthy after surgery.

Planning your meals is an important part of making the most of your food after surgery. If you plan your meals ahead of time, you can make sure you get a variety of nutrients throughout the day and not rely on fast foods that might not have enough of the nutrients you need. Take into account working with a trained dietitian to create a personalized meal plan that fits your dietary needs and tastes.

Along with planning your meals, using long-term wellness tips from experts can help you stay healthy after the recovery time is over. For example, these tips might include ways to deal with worry, stay active, get enough sleep, and practice mindfulness. Taking a whole-person approach to health can help your body heal and improve your health and vitality in the long run.

In conclusion, improving your diet after surgery is important for helping you recover and staying healthy in the long run.

Focusing on nutrient-dense foods, including healing recipes in your meal plans, and following long-term health tips from experts can speed up the healing process and help your body get stronger and thrive after surgery. You can get personalized advice and help on your way to better health and wellness by talking to a doctor or qualified dietitian.

CHAPTER 8
LONG-TERM NUTRITION AFTER RECOVERY

People who have had thyroid surgery, especially those who have had a thyroglossal duct cyst removed, need to make sure they have healthy eating habits that will last. When the thyroid gland or thyroglossal duct cyst is surgically removed, it can have a big effect on a person's food needs and health as a whole. Changing the way you eat after surgery is important for both your healing and your long-term health and wellness.

People often experience changes in their metabolic and hormonal balance after surgery, which can make it harder to control their weight and give them less energy. Focusing on nutrient-dense foods that help the metabolism work, speed up the mending process, and give you long-lasting energy is very important.

For long-term health and recovery after surgery, it's important to eat a balanced diet with lean proteins, complex carbohydrates, healthy fats, and a wide range of fruits and veggies. Proteins are needed to heal tissues and keep the immune system working well, and carbs give the body energy.

Healthy fats, like those in nuts, eggs, and olive oil, help your body make hormones and absorb vitamins that dissolve in fat.

Also, eating a range of fruits and vegetables makes sure that you get enough of the vitamins, minerals, and antioxidants that your body needs to work properly and repair damaged tissues. Because they are high in nutrients, dark leafy greens, berries, citrus fruits, and cruciferous veggies are especially good for you.

Getting plenty of water throughout the day is also important to stay fresh.

Staying hydrated helps the body digest food, absorb nutrients, and run cells normally, which leads to faster healing and recovery.

Along with eating nutrient-dense foods, developing sustainable eating habits includes mindful eating techniques like recognizing when you are hungry or full, controlling your portions, and not eating when you are upset. Mindful eating can help you avoid overeating and develop a good relationship with food, which can help you keep a healthy weight and a balanced diet over time.

Planning and making meals can also help people keep up healthy eating habits by making sure that healthy snacks and meals are always available. When people plan and make their meals ahead of time, they don't have to rely on fast foods that are often high in processed foods, bad fats, and added sugars.

Also, getting help from medical professionals like registered dietitians or nutritionists can give you personalized advice and education on how to improve your food and lifestyle based on your needs and goals. Working with a healthcare professional can help people make changes to their diet, fix nutrient deficiencies, and improve their health and wellness in the long run.

Overall, making lasting changes to the way you eat after thyroid surgery is important for speedy healing, long-term health and wellness, and eating a balanced diet. People can form healthy habits that improve their health and well-being by focusing on nutrient-dense foods, practicing mindful eating, and meal planning, and getting help from medical experts.

Food suggestions to help you live a healthy life

To stay healthy after having thyroid surgery, especially if a thyroglossal duct cyst was removed, you need to pay special attention to what you eat to help your body heal and stay healthy in the long run. Even though the first few days after surgery are very important for healing, following nutritional advice every day can help people do well and avoid problems in the future.

Making sure you get enough iodine is one of the most important health things to think about after thyroid surgery. Iodine is needed for the thyroid gland to make thyroid hormones, which are very important for controlling metabolism, growth, and development. Iodized salt and enriched foods give most people in developed countries enough iodine. However, people who are having thyroid surgery may need to keep an eye on their iodine levels and possibly take a supplement if they are not getting enough.

Calcium is another important nutrient to pay attention to. The parathyroid glands and the thyroid gland work together to control the body's calcium levels. Some people who have had surgery on their thyroid may end up with hypocalcemia, which means their calcium levels are too low.

So, eating foods that are high in calcium, like dairy products, leafy greens, and fortified plant-based milk replacements, can help keep your bones healthy and keep you from getting problems related to low calcium levels.

Also, it's important to keep an eye on your vitamin D levels because they are linked to bone health and calcium absorption. Vitamin D levels can be kept at a healthy level by getting enough sunlight and eating foods like fatty fish, fortified dairy products, and mushrooms that are high in vitamin D.

In addition to certain nutrients, people who have had thyroid surgery should focus on eating a balanced diet with a range of whole foods to make sure they get enough vitamins, minerals, and antioxidants. Meals that include lean proteins, complex carbohydrates, healthy fats, and lots of fruits and veggies can give you the nutrients you need to stay healthy and happy.

Also, watching your portions and practicing careful eating can help people stay at a healthy weight and avoid problems like weight gain or obesity, which can make thyroid-related conditions worse.

To avoid overeating, it's best to pay attention to your body's signals when you're hungry or full, watch your portions, and avoid mindless snacks.

Adding regular physical exercise to your daily routine is another important part of living a healthy life after thyroid surgery. Not only does exercise help you lose weight and keep your heart healthy, but it also improves your general health by lowering your stress, making you feel better, and giving you more energy.

Finally, keeping hydrated by drinking lots of water throughout the day is very important for digestion, hydration, and cell function in general.

It's especially important to stay hydrated after surgery to help the body heal and avoid problems like nausea or dehydration.

living a healthy life after thyroid surgery means paying attention to certain nutritional factors, such as getting enough iodine, calcium, and vitamin D. It also means putting an emphasis on a balanced diet, controlling portions, regular physical exercise, and staying hydrated. By using these nutrition tips every day, people can help their bodies heal better, avoid complications, and stay healthy in the long run.

CONCLUSION

The journey to optimal nutrition after surgery isn't just about getting better right away; it's also about being healthy in the long run. We've gone through the complete guide to the best post-surgery diet and talked about important topics like getting ready for surgery and keeping up healthy habits after healing.

Because we know how important nutrition is for recovery, we've put together a plan that starts with making your kitchen a healing space and then moves on to exploring healthy recovery foods that are perfect for each stage of recovery. Every recipe has been carefully chosen to help your body heal. They range from comfortable soups and smooth purees to tasty treats that change the texture of food and flavorful blended meals.

We've also stressed how important it is to have meals that are easy to swallow and give you a wide range of choices, from soft casseroles to delicate seafood dishes, so that your nutritional needs are met without sacrificing taste or texture. We've also added healthy snacks and treats to help you stay energized and avoid cravings while you're getting better.

Our guide goes beyond healing to include long-term nutrition, focusing on long-term eating habits and giving nutritional advice for living a healthy life.

Focusing on nutrient-dense foods and building muscle with meals that are high in protein helps us not only recover but also stay strong and healthy.

In the end, this complete guide is a lighthouse of support for people who are recovering from surgery. It includes not only healing foods and meal plans but also health tips for the long term.

As you start this trip, may you find nourishment, strength, and vitality that will help you have a better and healthier future.

www.ingramcontent.com/pod-product-compliance
Lightning Source LLC
Chambersburg PA
CBHW060800260726
48660CB00002B/705